Busy Mum Syndrome

How to Keep on Top of Your Health and Happiness

Kelly Rennie

Copyright 2016

Copyright © *Kelly Rennie*

ALL RIGHTS RESERVED. No part of this report may be reproduced or transmitted in any form whatsoever, electronic, or mechanical, including photocopying, recording, or by any informational storage or retrieval system without express written, dated and signed permission from the author.

DISCLAIMER AND/OR LEGAL NOTICES: The information presented in this report represents the views of the publisher as of the date of publication. The publisher reserves the rights to alter and update their opinions based on new conditions. This report is for informational purposes only. The author and the publisher do not accept any responsibilities for any liabilities resulting from the use of this information. While every attempt has been made to verify the information provided here, the author and the publisher cannot assume any responsibility for errors, inaccuracies or omissions. Any similarities with people or facts are unintentional.

CONTENTS

ABOUT THE AUTHOR 1
INTRODUCTION 5
WHY THIS BOOK IS DIFFERENT 7
THE PROBLEM WITH MODERN LIVING 13
BUSY MUM SYDROME DEMYSTIFIED 19
HOW TO HAVE THE BODY AND LIFE YOU DESERVE 24
NUTRITIONAL MISTAKES YOU NEED TO STOP MAKING 33
EXERCISE MISTAKES YOU NEED TO STOP MAKING 43
THE TIME ILLUSION – WHY THERE IS ALWAYS ENOUGH TIME 55
HOW TO SET GOALS YOU CAN ACTUALLY ACHIEVE 65
BREAKING NEGATIVE PATTERNS 75
THE MINDFULNESS SECRET: WHAT IT IS, HOW IT WORKS AND HOW TO GET STARTED 85
BRINGING IT ALL TOGETHER 95
WOULD YOU DO ME A FAVOUR? 98

ABOUT THE AUTHOR

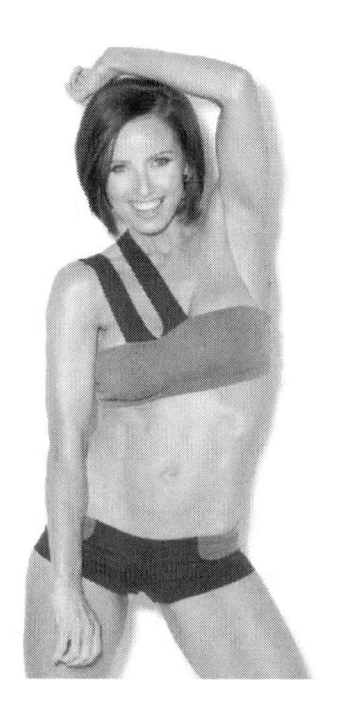

Hi I'm Kelly. My mission as a coach and personal trainer is to help you envision the body of your dreams, then encourage you to do what it takes to get it. I believe that with the right support anybody can take control of their health and fitness, enjoying an energy-filled, disease-free life in the process.

WHY YOU SHOULD TRUST ME

My health and fitness journey began in the beautiful country of New Zealand where, as a girl, I developed a passion for exercise and sport. Throughout my childhood I practiced gymnastics and kickboxing, as well as playing rugby and exercising on a daily basis. I didn't know it at the time but these early experiences planted the seeds for my future success.

I left New Zealand for the United Kingdom, where I ended up living for 10 years. For a long time I had no idea what I wanted to do. Things weren't great and I was continually haunted by the feeling that somehow I wasn't living up to my potential. My health also took a battering, suffering from chronic anxiety and depression.

That all changed on May 5th, 2010.

I remember the date precisely because it was the day I chose to take control of my life. Sitting in my local coffee shop I decided there and then to write a list of goals I would try my hardest to achieve. One of these goals was to compete in a physique contest. The very next day I acted on my goal and found a local trainer who had bodybuilding experience. They agreed to train me and I entered myself into the Natural Figure Bodybuilding Competition.

After 4 months of hard training and a dedicated eating routine I placed 3rd in the UK in the Figure Division of the British Natural Body Building Federation. Not long after this initial success I became a sponsored athlete with Optimum Nutrition in the UK and Designer Physique in Australia.

In December 2010 I went on to win the overall World Sports Model Agency Competition. In 2011, I was yet again in the BNBF Britain finals.

One thing led to another and my dedication to health and fitness has paid off a thousand times over. I'm became one of UK's top fitness models. I've worked with some of the biggest companies in the fitness world, such as bodybuilding.com, Oxygen Magazine, Muscle & Fitness and Optimum Nutrition. I'm was also the owner of two successful Prime Mover gyms, which are fast becoming known as Sheffield's #1 fitness and fat loss centres.

A lot has changed over the last few years. I'm now the Mummy of two gorgeous daughters, Nevaeh and Eden, who bring me more joy than I could ever have imagined. Having two kids in two years brought to the table a whole new lifestyle and systems to cope with life which I can't say I found that easy at the start. In 2014 we moved to the Gold Coast of Australia. It's from here that I put my experience together to create my online fitness business, helping thousands of Busy

Mums to transform their bodies and minds just like I did.

I'm proud to say that my credentials now include:

International Fitness Model & Athlete
Optimum Nutrition Athlete
Author "The Fit Mummy Manual"
Writer www.bodybuilding.com
Writer for New Zealand Fitness Magazines

Cover-girl for Leading Fitness Publications

Monthly contributor to Australian Oxygen Magazine
Pre and Post Natal Expert

How did all this happen?

If my experiences have taught me anything over the last 10 years it's that hard work really pays off. I never, ever stopped believing in myself and made it a constant discipline to write short and long-term goals that had to be completed within a certain timeframe. Staying focused and positive have allowed my dreams to come true before my eyes and I am grateful beyond words.

The best bit?

If I can do it so can you!

Looking forward to hearing about your success as you apply what you learn in this book!

Kelly Rennie xx

INTRODUCTION

Stop for a moment today and take a look around.

Busy mums, juggling home and work life, rushing to their next appointment. Wives pushing prams. Everywhere, constant and sometimes frantic movement. In the modern world we have become slaves to our smartphones and 'to do' lists, both of which hardly ever stop, leaving us wondering at the end of the day where all of the time went. Where all of our good intentions and goals fit into this frenetic, sometimes confusing, daily grind.

If you are anything like me the day starts before the sun comes up and ends long after it has gone down. With two young children to look after and a growing business to run there hardly seems to be enough time to eat, let alone work on my personal goals of better health and fitness. Sometimes it's like life doesn't want us to be in shape and to enjoy all of the great things that entails!

On the surface it looks like an impossible job. Especially when you look at all of the health and fitness 'rules' that get spouted about – long exercise sessions, marathon cardio, meal prep, an almost religious dedication to the cause. Then you get all of the celebrity 'secrets' that amount to nothing substantial, or realistic. It's enough to make anyone give up on the first day. We've got enough to do. Adding another huge commitment to the pile seems counter-intuitive somehow.

Well, I'm here to tell you that it can be done. You don't need to abandon your dream of having a fit, toned body that you can show off and be proud of. You don't have to cut short playtime with your kids. In fact, despite what magazines and celebrities with paid endorsements will tell you, it's the complete opposite.

The fact is you CAN get in healthy and fit on a tight schedule. You CAN still enjoy the foods you like without ruining your goals. You CAN maintain your fit frame with hardly any effort, in as little as fifteen minutes a few times a week.

WHY THIS BOOK IS DIFFERENT

I made a bold promise in the last section and it's ok to be sceptical. We've been led up the primrose path before. If you're like me, perhaps lots of times. It seems like there is always a new book, study or piece of research coming out which debunks the findings of the previous lot. It is a never-ending stream made murky by the fact that a lot of the 'health and fitness 101' rulebook that we have come to unconsciously accept was paid for by companies trying to sell their products. There are also a lot of clever marketers out there who know how desperate we are for a solution and will happily provide us with one, even though the results we were told to expect never quite materialise in the way that we hope.

I'm not ashamed to admit that, back in my early days, I fell for a lot of it. I would work out for hours at a time, would prep meals religiously. Almost all of my thoughts centred on the next workout, the next competition or photoshoot. Then, one day, all of that changed. I had two young children to look after and my days weren't quite as easy to navigate. For once, my own health and fitness would have to take a backseat. With two little people dependent on you long, intense workouts and strict dieting start to look less and less appealing, and less feasible.

Does this sound like you? If you are anything like the hundreds of clients that I have worked with over the years' then it will resonate on some level. It might not be children. It might be your career, your studies, or caring for an elderly relative that takes up the bulk of your time.

Becoming a busy mum with children and a career was a huge wake-up call. All of a sudden I had to evaluate all of the belief systems that had accumulated about health and fitness. About what it meant to me and what really worked. For the first time ever I was in the position where I had to question the dogma and rules that stop a lot of busy people from pursuit their fitness dreams. It was find a new way or forget about it.

Over the course of a few years I was my own test guinea pig. Exercises, diets, mind-sets, philosophies – it all came under the microscope. Having already had success in the fitness model world it was a tough thing to do. It was hard to let go of an identity and a set of values that had been so significant in my life. Thankfully it was a necessity so I persevered.

Over time I discovered a whole new set of rules and values that would work for any busy mum. I also discovered what is labelled here as 'Busy Mum Syndrome', which is really a catchy term for the negative spiral we find ourselves in when it feels like the clock is running our lives. It is what happens when our day-to-day living is out of balance, and it has far-reaching consequences on our overall physical, mental and emotional health.

This book is a condensed record of everything I learned and still practice to this day. Instead of spending years doing trial and error on various workouts and diets you can go directly to the goal of optimum health and fitness, tweaking things to fit in with your unique life situation as you go. What could be better than that?

Together, we'll find out:

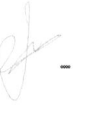

- The problem with modern living and why we find it so hard to put aside time for ourselves

- The reasons why 'Busy Mum Syndrome' has become such a prevalent menace in our society

- How to prepare to have the body and life you deserve

- Nutritional mistakes that are costing you time and that toned stomach

- Workout mistakes that are wasting time and not getting the results you want

- How to get time on your side and start winning at life

- How to complete a goal-setting process that you can actually stick to

- How to break negative patterns that are stopping you from progressing

- The mindfulness secret- why an ancient practice can increase your quality of life a hundred times over

- Why we are all in this together and how we can continue to help each other after we are done here

I know how busy you are and this might look like a lot of work but, trust me, it's worth it. When you have the specific, tested principles that will get you in shape and keep your mind sharp in the midst of your daily routine it will prove itself as a great investment in your future happiness.

So let's get to it. There's no time to waste.

THE PROBLEM WITH MODERN LIVING

There are so many advantages to living now. In developed countries food and hygiene is better than ever before. We can talk to people on the other side of the world at the press of a button, for nothing. There are gyms and health stores on every corner and long-distance travel is cheaper than at any other point in history, making it easier for us to discover and explore. On the surface most things are great. Scratch a little, however, and the glossy veneer starts to come away.

We as a species are overstressed, overworked and out of control emotionally, much of which is down to our modern environment. The one big problem with modern living is that we are always on the go, reacting rather than creating, at the beck and call of constant external stimuli like smartphones and media outlets. How many hours a day do we spend staring at screens? Even for the casual user it averages out at a couple of hours. For the office worker it can reach an eye-watering sixteen hours of screen-based focus, sometimes even more.

More than half of all working adults (yes, that's ALL) say they are concerned with the amount of stress in their lives. Sixty per-cent of people in poor health report having high stress levels. Many take potentially harmful drugs to combat this, most of which will only mask the symptoms and exacerbate the problem over time.

These stats clearly indicate that there is a huge issue with the way we live our lives. No one is particularly happy. Despite all of the material advantages of living right here and right now levels of contentment are at a low, and getting lower. What is it about being on the go that plagues us so much? Aren't we a species born to move quickly, to evolve, to spot opportunities and overcome challenges?

The crux of our worldwide problem can be found in our conception of time. Simply put, we feel like we don't have enough of it. On the rare occasion we feel like we have an abundance of time we are usually too frazzled, or too worried about something, to use it constructively.

From my own experience as a young mother I have seen this outwardly manifest as Busy Mum Syndrome. It is a pervasive menace. I have not met a young mum – whether family member, friend or client - who does not suffer from it to some degree. Going deeper you could say that it is a state of constant stress, the feeling that you 'should' be doing something else that gnaws at your stomach whilst you work. Over time it develops into a general feeling that you don't have control, that your life is on autopilot and there is nothing you can do about it. This leads to a progressive erosion of self-esteem and confidence in your own abilities. Personal goals go out of the window. Health and fitness, if it didn't exist in your life before, becomes something you see and read about but never do.

It is one of the saddest things not to achieve the goals you have set for yourself. It is even worse when you feel that they are beyond your control. Busy Mum Syndrome strips you of your right to choose by convincing you that all of the choices are already made. Once you readily accept this the only way is down; into a mire of depression, despondency, and vanishing willpower.

From the many mums I have spoken to about this there is one universal effect of BMS that we all suffer from – fatigue. The feeling that our energy is blocked or inhibited in some way, which causes functioning in the world to be an uphill battle. When we feel fatigued the last thing most of us want to do is hit the squat rack or pound some miles on the treadmill. The majority of comfort food is brought and ingested when we are in these lower emotional states, which only takes us further away from our desired figure, and another summer covering up.

There are actually scientific reasons why we feel this way, the main ones we will cover in the following chapter. Once we know what and why things are happening we can plot how to break the cycle. Bit by bit we can dig ourselves out and feel the sun on our faces again. We will also do this as we go on.

As for right now there is one thing you can do that will make the whole process a lot easier. That is to take a step back, away from your life story and that seemingly uncontrollable stream of events, and realise that time is abundant. Our stresses are merely a learnt reaction to our life situation and not knowing how to get the most out of what we already have. After this journey together you will never hear yourself say you haven't got time to be in shape again.

Modern life is so easy we have grown accustomed to having everything handed to us on a plate. If it isn't instant we are rarely interested, which makes optimal health and fitness a big dilemma.

We all want to look better. We all want more shapely legs, a toned stomach, a good bum and better skin. There is no shame in admitting it. These things are natural and a beautiful expression of our inherent potential and desire to unfold. The only issue is that the body is a slow mover. It can't be changed overnight. It especially can't be changed when the mind it is attached to is confused and distracted. This is like coming into a football match on the losing team. There is a big chance that any impact you make will be swallowed up by what has gone before. Habits and ingrained behaviours are hard things to change. That doesn't mean, however, that it can't be done.

For five minutes today stop and look around. Begin to take responsibility for yourself and your long-held goals. This is the beginning of the end of Busy Mum Syndrome in your life.

BUSY MUM SYDROME DEMYSTIFIED

A lot of the symptoms of Busy Mum Syndrome are the products of our hormones. When we get into a negative spiral our body's chemistry and autonomous nervous system fall out of balance, leading to many of the undesirable issues we touched on in the previous chapter.

The main culprit in all of this is cortisol, commonly known as the 'stress' hormone. In scientific terms it is known as a corticosteroid hormone and is released by the adrenal gland when we find ourselves in a stressful situation. In normal functioning stress isn't meant to last very long and the cortisol that has been released will begin to dissipate when the immediate threat has disappeared. When you are overstressed, however, or over-stimulated, large amounts of cortisol remain present in your brain and body for long periods of time. Over time this wears out our body-mind system, resulting in damage to the hippocampus, which plays a key role in the creation of memories.

There are a whole host of other negative effects that have their source in cortisol imbalance. One of the most noticeable is our susceptibility to changes in bodyweight. Many leading health professionals agree that people with consistently high cortisol levels are liable to carry excess fat around the neck, face and stomach areas. High blood pressure and hyperglycaemia can also result from too much cortisol flooding into the brain.

Apart from unstable bodyweight, high levels of cortisol flowing through the bloodstream can adversely affect the condition of our skin, causing it to appear thin or to bruise easily. Because of bodyweight and skin fluctuations stretch marks can develop, as can increased pigmentation in the knees and elbows.

On top of this we find ourselves in perpetually fatigued state. This is due to the key role that cortisol plays in our sleeping and waking cycles. As soon as we go out of balance excessive tiredness and lack of energy flow is almost a certain side-effect. There is also evidence to suggest that higher levels of cortisol make us weaker and make it more likely we will lose muscle tissue and bone density, none of which are going to help us if enhanced health and fitness is our goal.

Before we begin demonising cortisol, however, it is important to understand that it does have some positive effects. When allowed to come and go freely it is a natural part of our 'fight or flight' mechanism, which has kept humanity alive for thousands of years. In normal doses it can give us a quick burst of energy when needed, it can increase our immunity, lower our sensitivity to pain and help maintain homeostasis in the body. The enemy, then, is not really cortisol. It is our sedentary, stimulant-fuelled lifestyles and the way we react to the situations that arise.

Chronic stress and the consistent release of corticosteroids into the brain has been termed the 'silent killer' in recent years. Studies have shown that it can take ten years from your life and you won't ever know about it. Pretty distressing, right? Fortunately, there are a few things we can do that will significantly reduce the presence of stress in our lives. As we do so we will automatically see a huge improvement in our appearance, fitness levels and overall peace of mind. We will go over all of them in the following chapters.

As for right now a happy thought is that the #1 way to cut out stress is to participate in regular physical activity. It is a way for us to tap into our inherited 'fight' response in a constructive way, allowing us to release pent up anger and frustrations in the process. On a hormonal level this aids in burning up any excess cortisol that is floating around our system, greatly reducing our stress response when we are engaged in other areas of life. Just 15-20 minutes of semi-intense activity every couple of days will go a long way to enhancing our sense of wellbeing.

Aside from the obvious benefit for the body, regular physical activity will also aid the 'mental side' of the game. In this day and age much of our stress is mind-made. We rarely face physical dangers or threats to our lives so the mind compensates by getting stressed at other things. This makes mastering your mental response to stress very important.

Developing the willpower to make time and train hard will increase our self-confidence over time, which will in turn limit the presence of fear in our daily lives. Fear is the antithesis of what is positive in our existence. It tells us we can't do this or that, or that we aren't good enough. To build resilience in the face of fear, usually manifesting as hardships, brings about the realisation that we can handle whatever life throws at us. As this realisation dawns on us we find that there is a natural decrease in negative feelings, with a corresponding increase in positive feelings. Our daily lives become infinitely smoother. We sleep easier. The people we care about notice the change and respond to us in kind. Instead of being a slave to Busy Mum Syndrome, enduring a downward spiral, we are now spiralling upwards, positively affecting everything around us. As our actions are positively reinforced by the feelings we receive and the encouragement we get from the people around us, suddenly finding time to exercise is no longer an issue. Eating right just seems to happen as we now no longer feel the need to fill an emotional hole with sugar snacks or binge eating. Life becomes what it was always meant to be.

Think this sounds too good to be true? Ask anyone who takes their health and fitness seriously and makes it a priority in their day. I will bet big they say it changed their life. It can do the same for you.

HOW TO HAVE THE BODY AND LIFE YOU DESERVE

It might seem farfetched right now but you absolutely can have the body and life you deserve. The body you have dreamed about for years and pictured on a white sandy beach a million times. The life and lifestyle that minimises your stress and allows you to be productive and positive throughout your day. It's completely possible and can be yours faster than you can imagine. You just have to know what you are doing and how you block the good things from manifesting in your life.

If you are anything like I was there is always a persuasive reason not to take action, or gamble on something that may or may not pay off. These reasons always seem like the sensible, safe path and we justify them by telling ourselves we are just being realistic or it wouldn't have worked anyway. One of my favourites when putting the brakes on pursuing a dream is that 'it is probably for the best'.

For many of us, excuses run our lives. Whenever a remarkable opportunity or idea appears in our consciousness – which they do, don't be so modest – a corresponding, familiar voice pipes up simultaneously and guides us back to the status quo. Ever wonder why there are only a handful of people who look fantastic, or make lots of money, or work their dream careers? It's because of excuses. Listening to them and, even worse, believing them, is the death knell for any chance of success in any endeavour.

Excuses are infinite in variety and persistent by nature. They come when you least want them to and always hit you where it hurts, robbing you of your personal power. Some of the most common excuses include 'I'm too young', 'I'm too old', 'I don't have enough time', 'I don't have enough money', 'I'll do it when the kids are older', 'it's too risky', 'nobody will support me' and, the king of them all, 'I'm not good enough'. Do any of these sound familiar to you?

These, and thousands of other excuses like them, are why you don't have the body and life you deserve. When the time came to take action you fell back, listened to that whisper in the back of your head and gave up before you even got started. You might have even got quite far and then given up, which is actually even more painful. Whatever your story the excuses have shaped it in a way that you don't want. They are the ink blots on the page and it is time to erase them.

Before you can do this effectively you have to make a 100% commitment to do so. Listen to your mind for any period of time and you realise just how slippery it is. It likes the way things are and it absolutely does not want to change. It will resist your best intentions before even know it. You have to know and accept yourself intimately and be ready for the bumps in the road once the mind gets an idea of what you are attempting to do.

When it comes to exercise there are generally five excuses that everybody experiences. Of course, there are others but many of these are personal and have their roots in poor self-image. After talking to hundreds of mums the five general excuses are pretty much a human-wide experience. After all, our brains aren't that much different. We all have the same in-built defence mechanisms that try and preserve the status quo instead of attempting something new.

Some of these excuses we have touched on before but they are: 'I don't have time, 'I'm too tired', 'I can never get away from the kids', 'exercise is boring' and 'I've tried before and got nowhere'. Trust me, if you are new to all of this you are going to hear these in your head quite often, at least until you ingrain exercise as a positive lifestyle habit that you are better off keeping. Let's look at each one in turn and 'de-fang' them, so when they do crop up they will have lost all of their persuasive power.

1) I don't have enough time

By far the most common excuse as to why people can't hit their fitness goals, 'I don't have enough time' has been around as long as people have cared about what they look like (forever). On the surface it sounds like an insurmountable challenge – we only have so much time, right? Go a little deeper, however, and take an unbiased look at how you really spend your days. What you will find is that 'finding time' for exercise (and anything you struggle to fit in) is simply a matter of prioritisation. We will touch on this in much more detail in a later chapter.

2) I'm too tired

Ask anyone who has hit the gym after a bad day, when they didn't feel like this could do it – exercising actually made them feel better! The energy boost from vigorous activity is no placebo, either. Exercise causes the body to release a plethora of 'feel good' hormones, or endorphins, which help curb fatigue and significantly enhance your mood. The fact is most of the tiredness we experience is just a sign of emotional withdrawal; by the end of the day we want to escape ourselves and the day so the mind-made tiredness prepares us for the oblivion of sleep. When this happens flip the switch to something positive and force yourself to exercise anyway. Within minutes you will be in the flow of the exercise, your blood will be pumping and you will feel much better. The natural high will last long after the workout has finished, too.

3) I can never get away from the kids

Many of the mums that I know, including myself, have really struggled with this one. It seems like a hopeless endeavour to try and snatch away half an hour for exercise when we have a little person dependent on us. Combined with the idea that 'exercise is boring' this is usually enough to kill off any dream body aspirations forever. It certainly was for me until I realised that the kids are not an obstacle to health and fitness, they are actually an aid! Doing activities with your kids, such as cycling or jump rope, can help them as much as it helps you. Not only will you improve your health and enhance your mother-child bond, it will also instil a positive habit in your children that will serve them well in later life.

4) Exercise is boring

There are so many reasons why this isn't true! For many people who believe that exercise is boring it is because they have been introduced to an activity that doesn't suit them. Hour long cardio sessions aren't for everybody. Some people like to do weights in the gym, or bodyweight circuits in their living room. Others like sport, or dance, or training with others as part of a social group. The variety of exercise is endless. Go with your heart on this one and never be afraid to try something new, if it appeals. Making the body-mind healthier is a natural activity and there is something for everyone.

5) I've tried before and got nowhere

So many people have tried and failed to get their health and fitness in check. Almost every home that I have been in has, or once had, a 'graveyard' of gimmick exercise machines and a stack of barely opened nutrition books. Exaggerated promises and deceptive marketing practices have turned our dreams into ashes more times than we care to remember. All of this has left a bad taste in our mouths and so exercise has been filed away in our minds as an unpleasant experience not worth repeating. Well, now it's time to try again! Things will be different this time. The key is to be realistic with the goals you set yourself. Set simple, achievable goals that you can knock out routinely. This will perk up your confidence and get some real momentum going. Later on we will talk about how to set small, manageable goals that lead to massive results over time.

When you learn to effectively cut off these excuses before they gather momentum you will have gone a long way to succeeding at your fitness goals. The same practice can be used for life goals, too. Simply identify the dominant excuses that apply to a certain area of your life and 'de-fang' them. See and understand clearly why they are false and do not help you at all. Once the excuses have been handled success will be easier and faster than you thought possible.

A Note on the 'Comfort Zone'

Almost all of us want a passionate, fearless life full of love and energy. We want to look great and to feel even better but we take no steps to achieving it. When we sell ourselves out like this the price is a consistent erosion of self-esteem and a gradual withdrawal from all of the things we enjoy. Not expecting love and energy is one of the secret root causes of social anxiety, a debilitating mental issue which stops many people from living fulfilled lives. In the end we get entrenched in what has been called the 'comfort zone', a seemingly safe place where everything is predictable and nothing risky ever happens.

This is all well and good for a while but one price of remaining in this place is that our personal growth stagnates and eventually stops. The fearful thoughts and emotions that caused you to retreat back into the comfort zone in the first place do not leave you. In fact, they grow stronger as time passes. Your indefinite retreat from the challenges of life feeds them indefinitely. Over time you suddenly realise you now fear failure, you fear the disapproval of others, and you especially fear the idea of trying anything new. Before you may have only been bothered by one of these things. This regression, when noticed, comes as a shock and deep feelings of dissatisfaction begin to creep in. It turns out that the comfort zone is not all that was promised. That by selling yourself short you have actually created what you feared most in the first place.

The comfort zone goes hand in hand with the symptoms of busy mum syndrome. Unless you fully commit to step out of it and take some short-term discomfort in the process of achieving your goals the whole thing becomes a lost cause. If you do commit amazing things will be on their way to you. Personal growth will resume, fears will disappear, regret will become excitement and the restrictions of the past become nothing more than a laughable story. Only when the comfort zone is far behind in the distance do you get a chance at the body and life you deserve.

What will you choose?

NUTRITIONAL MISTAKES YOU NEED TO STOP MAKING

There is a lot of misinformation out in the fitness world, especially about diet and nutrition. For every new diet or superfood there are ten others ready to take its place over the coming months. It can get really confusing, which will crush your motivation before you even begin. It's important to find what works for you and then drown out the rest of the noise ruthlessly. Trust me, there is always a better workout or better diet that you could be trying, which will only have you starting from scratch every few weeks and spinning your wheels endlessly.

One thing that is true is that 70% of our results will come from the foods we eat. You may have heard the phrase 'abs are made in the kitchen'. From my own experience, for the most part, I can say that this is correct. In order to get the most from our bodies on a daily basis we need to fuel them with the most nutrient-dense, efficient foods we can buy. Though this can be difficult to begin with it gets much easier over time, especially when the results you've always wanted start flooding in faster than ever! Before long you can't even remember how you used to eat or why you used to do it. Junk food loses its appeal when you realise it does nothing for you or your goals. Your new habits and success are then with you for life.

To get you started on the road to healthier eating and to supercharge your immediate progress there are a few nutritional mistakes that you should know about. Many of them will appear as common sense as you read them but you would be surprised how many people don't pay attention, or worse, turn a blind eye to their own actions. Committing to memory and refusing to make these mistakes will put you in the top ten per cent of people who are ready to take control of their health and fitness.

Ready? Let's get started.

1) Not reading the food label

We've mentioned how unscrupulous the marketing can be in the fitness industry but it can be just as bad for everyday household items, such as food. The hard truth is that a lot of food companies straight up lie about their product in order to shift more units. If lie seems like a strong word to you let's just say that they bend the truth a little, sometimes a lot, in order to tell the customer what they want to hear.

Perhaps the worst instance of this is the misleading information we sometimes find on food labels. Because top marketing agencies and businesses know that the average person doesn't know much about nutrition they can turn something that is clearly not good for you into something healthy-sounding. By adding small amounts of a certain ingredient they can boast that such and such product 'contains omega 3' or is 'low in fat', when really the main ingredients are sugar and flour. Even so-called health foods are guilty of this sometimes, especially dried fruits and preserved snacks.

Now that you know it is crucial you read the labels of the food you are buying. Look closely and make sure that what you are getting is not just a healthy-sounding cake. Train yourself to look past the promotional slogans and boasts. Remember that all of that is there to sell, not educate. Making this a habit will also ensure that you don't get demotivated when all of the 'health foods' you have brought aren't helping you towards your goals. Now you know why and can change course.

2) Skipping the protein

Everyone knows how important protein is by now, right? With the explosion in popularity for supplements and other health foods it's almost impossible to miss it.

With that said, health and nutrition authorities still recommend a relatively low daily protein intake. This might be ok if you are completely sedentary but for those of us who pursue an active lifestyle the amount advocated is simply too low for optimum health and performance. There are also many studies out there that definitively conclude that an increased protein intake can help to enhance overall body composition, especially if the person is physically active in some way.

If you need any more reasons to stop skipping protein know that it is also the most satiating macronutrient out of the bunch. This means you can keep your appetite suppressed for much longer over, say, a carb-focused meal. It also burns a significant amount of calories during the metabolic (digestive) process, helping you to burn more fat without any additional exercise!

Want a quick rule of thumb to live by for when you are in a rush? If in doubt, drop the carbs. Protein should always be the foundation of any meal if you want to be fit and healthy for the long-term.

3) Avoiding dietary fat

In the 1960s many of the most reputable nutritionists of the day concluded that the consumption of saturated fat was the number one cause of heart disease. When the theory gained traction in mainstream media the high-carb, low-fat diet came into popularity – and it has been with us in some form ever since.

It's only recently that new studies are showing that the consumption of dietary fat is not dangerous to your health at all. Fats actually raise your HDL cholesterol, which is the 'good' cholesterol, and transform the bad LDL cholesterol into something harmless. There is also lots of research to suggest that there is absolutely no correlation between the consumption of saturated fats and cardiovascular disease.

What does butter, eggs and fatty meat all have in common? They are all delicious and good for you! Forget what you have been told about fat and give it a leading role in your diet. You will be glad you did.

4) Relying on processed foods

It's a sad fact of life that as our knowledge of nutrition has grown our health as a species has sharply declined. Until a few decades ago the prospect of widespread obesity seemed ridiculous. Increases in heart disease, diabetes and other health-related illnesses would have been equally so.

There has been a lot of finger pointing as to why this has happened. Many suggest that is our increasingly sedentary lifestyles that have caused this. More than likely it is our poor food choices. Learning about calories, macros and vitamins has, in the whole, not really helped us at all. This is because as we were learning about these things there was a huge increase in the amount of processed and 'factory made' foods made available for our consumption. Loaded with trans fats and vegetable oils, these foods offered us three things we find hard to turn down – cheapness, abundance and instant gratification. It's no surprise that our health has greatly suffered as a result!

If you are serious about increasing your health and fitness levels it is time to get rid of the processed food habit. Prepare and eat real, natural foods that are full of nutrients and provide exactly what your body needs. If you are ever confused just ask yourself whether you would find what are eating in nature. If not, you can definitely do better.

5) Focusing too much on calories

It's easy to try and simplify a diet by saying that all that matters are calories. This way, we can still eat all of the 'bad' things that we want because, hey, that's all we've eaten today!

As much as I wish this was true, it's not. Even though calories are an important part of diet regulation they are not the only, or the most important, part. The truth is that different foods and macronutrients go through different metabolic pathways and so affect the body in a variety of ways. You didn't think that piece of cake and that bowl of spinach really went down the same way, did you?

Calorie counting can work as a method for portion control for certain people. Others, however, will find it easier to focus on better food choices than to get loaded down with numbers. It really comes down to the person but making solid food choices a habit is the effective way to go. Putting an emphasis on counting calories without checking what food is going in will just end in frustration when the weight stops coming off.

6) Believing that eating healthy is no fun!

The number one nutritional mistake that stops so many women from creating their dream body is the belief that eating healthy is a boring way to go. That all of the foods available are bland, unexciting and not worth the effort. There is even a widespread belief that eating healthy and avoiding large amounts of alcohol is a social life killer, which is an especially large issue for younger women. With so much pressure on body image these days it seems like a cache 22 situation – so I become fit and boring or unhealthy and interesting?

In reality eating healthy and being healthy does not have to be boring at all. Fresh, well-cooked meals consisting of non-processed foods will offer many of the best culinary experiences you can hope for. It is also a fantastic way to experiment and try new things – spices, sauces and other homemade extras can take what might seem like a bland meal to another level. Healthy eating doesn't have to take an age to prepare, either. You can usually cook something up in the time it takes to put a pizza in the oven. There are so many cookbooks out there now showing you how to be healthy whilst enjoying what you eat that the idea that you somehow have to become boring seems almost redundant. Haven't you heard? Fit is now fashionable.

The chances are high that you are guilty of some of the key nutritional mistakes above. We all are, whether now or at some time in the past. The main thing is to become fully aware of what we have been doing and to start the process of change as we sit here now. It will feel odd at first, somehow forced and unnatural, but this just indicates that you are on the right path. The mind is naturally resistant to change, no matter how positive that change might be. In many ways the mind has absolutely no idea what is good for it. Understand that and make a friend out of the little voice in your head. It will make all of this so much easier.

Many of us will find we are much more likely to make a nutritional mistake when we are in a rush. This is when we go on to autopilot and forget all of our good intentions just to make the immediate moment seem smoother and more under our control. Resist when this urge comes up within you. The short-term gratification will turn on you in a heartbeat once you realise you have compromised on your goals and given up some very hard-earned ground.

It will be helpful, in the long run, if you re-read this chapter several times over the next few weeks. This repetition will help you to integrate these new action principles into your life with less hassle. Many of these mistakes we have made for a good portion of our lives, maybe the whole of our lives, so they are not going to go away without a fight. You may even find yourself acting them out unconsciously several times before you start to snap out of it. Don't worry. Re-read when you can and remain vigilant when you are around food. Before long your diet, and body, will be unrecognisable and you won't even realise what happened.

EXERCISE MISTAKES YOU NEED TO STOP MAKING

Just like the nutritional mistakes in the previous chapter, there are a lot of ways we can go wrong with exercise. Many of these issues stem from bad advice and misinformation, cutting our results in half and making it less likely we will integrate fitness training into our lifestyle. You may have been here before – training, working hard, not really enjoying what you are doing, only to be disappointed by the end result. The chances are that one or more of the exercise mistakes below were being made on at least a semi-consistent basis.

Despite what most trainers say exercise should be approached as a very individual thing. Just as we all have different temperaments, our bodies respond differently to physical stressors. This is the main reason most exercise routines don't work out. We are actually pushing our bodies in a way that it isn't suited to, creating suboptimal results and leading us into a seemingly inescapable plateau. One we hit that glass ceiling exercise becomes a chore, not something to look forward to and progress at. You see this all of the time in the gym. Women plodding away on the treadmill or bicycle, completely zoned out reading a book or watching TV, trying to do everything they can not to fully experience where they actually are and what they are doing.

Then there's the fact we are so busy. "I don't have time" kills so many fitness aspirations. Most workouts you see online and in magazines require a substantial time commitment, which already sets up a losing game for the normal person. We need rules that are powerful and practical, something we can follow in complete faith that it will give us the results we want without having to get too bogged down in details and technicalities. This way we can step away from our exercise time refreshed and invigorated, reads to successfully deal with other parts of our hectic lives.

Cookie-cutter routines and programmes don't work as well as we'd like. We know that. There are, however, certain principles that we can learn that will give us the most 'bang for our buck' in the shortest amount of time. These you will figure out and integrate automatically as you recognise the exercise mistakes below. Cutting these out is going to blast your progress into the stratosphere. Then, as your motivation and momentum snowballs, you will see the positive and mental effects come back tenfold.

1) Picking the wrong type of exercise

So many people get demotivated when it comes to exercise because it doesn't deliver what it promises. Either that or it delivers something different to what was desired. You see it all the time in gyms. Someone hitting the weights hard when really all they want to do is increase their cardio. Likewise, someone else wanting to 'tone up' and spending hours on the treadmill, finally stopping and wondering where their great curves have gone.

The issue here is lack of awareness. Starting out, none of us have any idea what physical activity we may have an affinity for. We can read and learn but it really comes down to trial and error. I tried tons before I found what fit in with my goals and lifestyle. You need to ask what works for me? How can I get the largest return on the small amount of time I have to invest?

I can in no way tell you what type of exercise will work best for you and your unique life situation, let alone tell you what type of exercise you will most enjoy. I can only tell you what works for me. If you have a busy lifestyle, perhaps a few kids to look after, you may find it useful.

I employ a type of raining known as HIIT (High Intensity Interval Training). For me and many others it offers all of the muscle building, fat burning benefits of longer sessions, without the added time commitment. For those who are unfamiliar with the term, HIIT combines periods of high intensity exercise with periods of lower intensity, cycling them in strategic intervals to ensure max effort and recovery. Studies have shown that with workouts that are only four minutes long you can increase your athletic capacity, positively affect your body composition and even improve glucose metabolism. Learning the technique and putting everything into the workouts I perform has allowed me to maintain my figure whilst juggling a business, two kids and a pretty hectic lifestyle. If this sounds similar to your situation it can probably do the same for you!

2) Not having workout goals

Though exercise involves moving our bodies it is ultimately a mental game. To get the most from it you have to know how the mind works and how to get it to play ball. If you don't you will always stop short of your maximum potential and never find out what you were actually capable of.

In a nutshell, the mind is a goal-oriented machine. It needs to be working towards what it perceives as pleasurable experiences or it stagnates and withdraws. This can be very destructive from a personal and social perspective so it's important to not let it happen.

Exercise, because it causes a certain amount of discomfort, is not something the mind will favour unless it frames the pain as preceding something pleasurable. One of the easiest ways to do this it to set goals for each workout. Bodybuilders and elite athletes do this intuitively, always aiming for a better performance in the next workout, whether that means more weight lifted, more repetitions, or a faster sprint time. You must do the same thing. Either more repetitions in a certain exercise or less time between sets will work fine. This habit of consistently smashing self-imposed limitations will keep you on the edge and will keep your mind sharp. Exercise will then become a key part of your evolution into someone you always wanted to be.

Exercise without specific goals can never reach the heights that are possible. Don't fall into the trap that goals are just for the neurotic. They are a huge part of how the brain mechanism works and an unbelievably powerful force that you can get working for you right now.

3) You spend too much time on 'prep' exercises

One of the biggest traps you can fall into when training is fooling yourself you are working towards your goals when you are really not. The most common way we do this is by focusing excessively on warm ups and correction exercises. Another way is to put more time into learning the correct form of an exercise, rather than actually just performing the exercise! It sounds ridiculous but trust me it happens, more often than you think.

Correction exercises, such as those that help muscular imbalances, are great supplements to a programme, just as long as they aren't the whole programme. We all have slight imbalances and injuries but that shouldn't stop you from diving in and getting what you want from exercising. Too many people use 'corrective' and 'functional' routines in order to avoid doing the hard work. Make no mistake, depending on your starting point, it will be hard. Excuses, even cleverly disguised ones such as 'prep work', will only delay the inevitable. In the end, you only sell yourself short when you don't take on the challenge before you.

Key takeaway? Do the hard work now, with the time you have. Trust me, once you begin, you will find a way. Work on the other things (imbalances, niggling injuries, muscle aches) as and when they appear.

4) Warming up the wrong way

The traditional way to warm up is to use a series of static stretches to engage the muscles and to get ligaments/tendons ready for action. If you have exercised before there is a high probability that you have done something like this. We all have, right? Well, turns out we had it wrong the whole time. Warming up with static stretches is actually terrible for workout performance, especially if you are focusing on some kind of resistance training. They have been shown conclusively to reduce available strength and to significantly lower body stability, resulting in a severely impaired workout.

If you want to warm up in a way that won't impact your performance use dynamic stretches. This is a combination of active and static stretching that will prepare your muscles for the overload that is coming. After training you can then use the more traditional static stretches to help with any post-workout tightness. As with most things, the order in which we act is a key component to success.

5) Not listening to your body

The hands down biggest mistake you can make when exercising is not listening to your body. The body is a finely tuned, sensitive organism that generally knows what is best for it. If it didn't I doubt we would have survived as long as we have! As a modern, intellectual society we have gotten used to living from the 'neck up'. By this we mean we engage our thinking process for almost everything, neglecting the feelings and sensations that our body constantly feeds us. Look closely and you realise that those sensations are just as important as our thoughts, sometimes more so. Especially in a vigorous physical activity we need to be able to decipher what it is telling us.

The age-old motto for exercising is 'no pain no gain' but this isn't always true. We need to be able to differentiate between the pain of exertion and the pain of injury. You'd think it would be obvious but it is easy for the lines to get blurred. So many times I have pushed myself too far, injuring myself in the process and setting the achievement of my goals back by several weeks.

There is also the intuitive aspect to look at. Our feelings generally indicate something long before our logical minds have the opportunity to catch up and verbalise it, hence the expression 'listen to your gut'. It's important to develop the capacity to shut off your mind and to hear what your body is telling you. Many times this will lead you to push harder, beyond the mental limits that you had set for yourself, unaware that your body could do more. Sometimes it means simply backing off and living to fight another day. Remember that, as incredible as our brains are, they are inherently mechanical and cannot always tells what is good for the system as a whole.

Ask anybody who has reached a high level of success in a sport of physical task and they will tell you the same thing. In fact, ask anyone who has achieved success in any task. My bet is that listening to the whole of your body, and not just your mind, was a very important part of the process. Luckily for us, exercise is one of the best ways to use and grow this ability. Over time you will be so in-tune with the whole of your body-mind that you will know what needs to be done instantly.

Mistakes that we make when exercising are just part of a larger learning process that ultimately result in the attainment of our goals. As busy mums it's important that we cut this learning curve as short as possible, without compromising on the beneficial experience of trial and error. The way to do that is by engaging others who have already achieved what we want and learning from them. We don't actually have to fail at something personally before we can learn the hard-earned lessons of someone else.

It's a curious fact of life that when we want something desperately we actually block it from appearing in our lives. This isn't anything mystical or mysterious. It is simply a self-sabotaging facet of the mind that translates extreme 'want' as extreme 'lack'. By wanting more than anything to be fit and healthy we can sometimes fall prey to this sort of behaviour without even realising it. It manifests in many ways; changing workouts every couple of weeks, skipping sessions, working out when we know we are tired and probably not able to give our best, organising easy workouts that don't challenge us in the ways that we need to be challenged. By highlighting some of the mistakes we make we can cut off this possibility before it is even on the horizon, as many of these mistakes are elements of the very same self-sabotaging behaviour. Becoming aware of them will make it easy to separate real, positive action from time-filling (read: time-killing) activities.

Make a sincere effort to spot these mistakes in your own workout plans. If you haven't started exercising yet be ready for when they start to creep in. They will, and you need to be there to shut the door on them when they do.

THE TIME ILLUSION – WHY THERE IS ALWAYS ENOUGH TIME

If you have read this far thinking "this all sounds great Kelly but when do I have the time?" you are not alone. In the modern world, as busy mums with thriving careers and family lives, it does feel sometimes as though the clock is against us.

It's a fact of life that we often find ourselves rush around frantically, minds buzzing and bodies zig-zagging this way and that, doing all that we can but never quite feeling as though we have done enough. We find ourselves complaining, more often than not, about the lack of extra hours in the day. If we have just one more hour to ourselves, we reason, we could do it all. We could be who we really want to be.

After a while of this churn and burn lifestyle we inevitably crash, mentally and literally, on to the sofa. The constant mounting of tension finally gets to us and the clock ticks onwards. Finally, consumed by our guilt and sense of powerlessness, we get back up and resume the grind. Until next time, sofa.

The whole thing then starts to appear as a relentless and ruthless treadmill. We find ourselves buried in unrewarding busy work. Nothing that we truly, deeply value is accomplished in any meaningful way.

Happily, however, this rather depressing image is actually an illusion.

The truth is there have been times in your life when accomplishment has come easy to you. That, despite how busy you were and how stacked your timetable looked, you found the time to set clear goals and confidently move towards them. Many of us do this unconsciously when we really want something so don't worry if you can't remember right now. When you have a quiet moment later on, think back and you will see that it is true. The proof won't be hard to find because the mind naturally holds on to fond memories that can give us a feeling of pleasure upon recollection.

When you recognise this phenomenon in your life you will know intuitively how to achieve your desires, despite the apparent busyness of your schedule. You will see that, in the times we really wanted something, time seemed to magically reshuffle itself in order to accommodate our new intentions. The extra hours, minutes and seconds we needed to see it through were suddenly there, as though we were just waiting for a reason to use them.

This is the big thing we need to wrap our heads around. *There is always enough time to do everything we want.*

We learn this by setting our personal goals and taking assertive action in spite of everything else that is going on around us. If that means waking up an hour earlier or going to bed an hour later then so be it. If it means hitting the gym in your lunch hour or prepping meals on a Sunday evening, rather than watching the television, then so be it. Once we begin to live this way, without self-imposed constraints in relentless pursuit of our goals, we suddenly realise that time is actually on our side. Its inevitable march forward is just a constant reminder to begin where we are. To match its step and to keep moving in the right direction.

Time, physicists tell us, is actually an illusion. It is an artificial framework that begins and ends in the mind. Somewhere along the way the mind and time separated and became enemies. Bring them back together and reconcile them and you will achieve more than you ever hoped for.

There are three key ingredients for personal achievement when tied down by a heavy schedule:

1) Motivation

It all begins with a very strong desire to get what you want. If your desire is strong enough any obstacles in the way merely appear as momentary distractions. You aren't scared of failing because there is nothing out there that could possibly make you fail. Your resolve is so strong that time is not an issue.

Take losing weight, for example. You have a sincere, burning desire to get your pre-baby body back. It's so powerful that you find yourself naturally waking up before anyone in the house does, pumped up and ready to give your all to your chosen workout routine. By the time everybody else is awake and making their way downstairs to the kitchen you are done, showered and eating breakfast. To everybody else nothing has changed but to you everything has changed. From being rushed off your feet and having no direction you have just made more time out of nothing, by sheer force of will. With this sort of action-taking energy the goal of reclaiming your pre-baby body is not just probable, it is inevitable.

When your desire is not very strong it is almost impossible to bend time to your will. Anything and everything seems to be telling you that what you are attempting is stupid. Obstacles and time commitments spring out of nowhere, hitting you when you least expect them and delaying the assault on your goals time and time again. Nobody appears very supportive, even your close friends and family. One slightly negative response is enough to shut down operations for a week or so. As a result, you don't get up any earlier and you are always too tired at night to make any meaningful headway.

Let's look at our losing weight example again. As great as the intention is to get your pre-baby body back the lack of real desire you feel is going to stop it dead. You will continue to get up when everyone else does and will immediately be rushed off by the days' activities. The frequent image in your mind of your younger body makes you feel good but you know deep down that you don't have what it takes to get it back. There just isn't the time anymore.

Do you see the difference?

Having a burning, all-powerful motivating force within you is not be underestimated. It is the one master key that unlocks all of your goals, whether that is losing weight, toning up, or just improving your health. "But I don't have that!" you say. That's ok right now, don't worry. The truth is not many of us do when starting out with something new and challenging. The road ahead is too uncertain for us to be 100% confident. That doesn't matter as long as we have the steadfast intention to stay the course. Visualise your desired body as often as you can. See your workouts before you do them and imagine how good you will feel when you are done. Over time, the images you create in your mind will become sharper, until they are crystal clear. When that happens your motivation will skyrocket all of its own accord. There is a part of our mind that cannot differentiate between external reality and imagination. Use it to your advantage and step fearlessly into what you want.

2) Prioritisation

Prioritisation should spring naturally from your motivation to do a thing. It is the minds' way of reshuffling the day-to-day of our lives to make way for this new important event. If motivation is the emotional side of accomplishing a goal then prioritisation is the logical side, where we take one step at a time. This is where the rubber meets the road, so to speak, and where we start to gather real momentum. When we prioritise something we also affirm to ourselves that what we are attempting is completely possible. That we do, in fact, have plenty of time.

Our priorities in life should always reflect what we want to have, where we want to go and who we want to be. If, for example, we want to be the world's best mum (who doesn't?) then we should make sure to spend quality time with our children every single day, strengthening the love that we share with them. If we want to be a fitness model, we would prioritise our time in the gym and our time cooking healthy meals in line with our body goals. The mental reshuffle of prioritisation allows us to focus on what we want and need, filtering out any superfluous extras and putting them at the bottom of the pile.

Looking at our losing weight example again, look at what would happen if we consciously made it a priority in our lives. Suddenly those after-work drinks don't seem so important anymore. I don't really need a lie in, you find yourself saying on Sunday morning. Without even knowing it we are out of the blocks and already hurtling towards the finish line.

From my own experience having three priorities at any one time is the optimal amount we can handle. Two of those are non-negotiable, being family/friends and work. The other one is up to you but you stand the best chance of achieving it if you won't overload yourself with other things. For me, my third priority is my health and fitness. These three ensure I don't get side-tracked and end up wasting time on things that don't contribute to my long-term happiness.

3) Challenging yourself

It can be tough to take the jump and make a change in your routine. Upsetting the status quo is always unsettling to begin with, especially if you have other people dependent on you or used to things being a certain way. Don't let this stop you, however. Once you have a strong desire for something it is your given right to go after it with all material means at your disposal. To do less than that is to bring yourself down mid-stride and to never really see yourself at you best.

It will be a decision you may regret in the future, when you are older and looking back.

Real change is painful and takes time. Your motivation will need to be reinforced time and time again before you reach your destination. Priorities will have to be juggled as life throws unexpected things your way. Once or twice you might find yourself exercising in the middle of the night, when everybody else is asleep. That's ok. It's all part of the process of becoming who you want to be. You will be thankful you did it later. It will be a funny story that you can be proud of.

Commit right now to a health and fitness goal that you have always wanted to achieve. Imagine it vividly and feel the motivation flow through you. Organise your day so that time is on your side. Then come back and tell me when you succeed.

What we have spoken about in this chapter is nothing new. These are things that we all know but forget as we get busy and more stressed. Right now I want you to make an unwavering commitment to see your goal to completion. To start a daily plan that will bring it to you step by step, making you feel more alive in the process. Make a decision right now. You will know when you have. Time will bow down to your powerful commitment. It will show you just how possible it really is. That is what it is meant to do.

After a few weeks or months, the daily practice you initially had no time for will become a focal point of your day. It will have a gravitational force that pulls in your focus and dedication like a tractor beam. You see this all of the time in your social circle. People who apparently had no interest in weight training or playing the piano suddenly posting photos or videos of their progress so everyone can see. They have tapped into a powerful desire they have repressed for too long and are now reaping the rewards of their hard work. Once you have such singleness of purpose then come the results.

HOW TO SET GOALS YOU CAN ACTUALLY ACHIEVE

If you are anything like most people setting goals is not something that comes naturally to you. It's actually not something we do at all if we can help it, except when it comes to setting a few token new years' resolutions. And we all know how they went.

Why are we so resistant to setting goals and going after them? A lot of it comes down to the added pressure of accountability. Once we have written something down we have made a silent pact with ourselves to see it through, no matter what. This sense of disruption, of what it might do to established norms, is too much for most people, despite the fact the transition period is never as bad as imagined.

With all of the failed resolutions over the years it can be easy to get into the mind-set that goal setting doesn't work. It makes no difference, we complain. You can write things down all that you want. It doesn't mean they are going to happen.

Can't argue with that logic. The thing is though that goal setting does work. It's worked for millions of people across the world, over generations and for centuries, many of whom attained what they wanted and ended up living rich, fulfilling lives. Maybe it isn't goal setting itself that doesn't work. Maybe it's us. Maybe it's the way we approach it.

As we take control of our health and fitness it is a good time to get to grips with the art of goal setting. Forget all about half-hearted new years' resolutions. You won't need them anymore. Things are going to change in a big way. I promise that if you take the real process of goal-setting to heart you will be amazed at how far you've come when you look back in a years' time.

Before we begin it is important to know what goal setting really is. At its core it isn't about wanting to be able to run a marathon or to have six-pack abs, though they are both admirable aspirations. It is simply the process of discovering where and who you want to be, by diving deep into yourself. This idea alone is enough to stop most people from verbalising their goals, even to themselves. Not knowing where we want to be can sometimes feel liberating but, in general it is a sneaky way for most people to bypass the anxiety of potentially failing at something. Failure is painful but it is a lot better than setting off with no direction, for fear of what others might think, suddenly finding yourself years later miles from where you really wanted to go.

I hope that is enough to motivate you to set goals for yourself. It really is the best way to get something important done. It's cathartic in that we really have to open up to ourselves about what we want, after years of pushing it down. Some of the things that come up may surprise you. Being true to yourself in such an authentic way feels great and allows for a lot more energy to flow in the direction of your passions, where it really matters.

There is a simple framework that I use to set goals that are important to me. It doesn't have to be shiny and special and it isn't. It simply has to give you that push to get out of bed in the morning and to keep going.

1) Start with why

Everything big starts with why. The mind needs to find purpose in our goals, otherwise it will rebel against the discomfort we are subjecting it to. Starting with why is also one of the hardest things you can do. Many of us are used to doing things without purpose, or at least a purpose that is dear to us. Be honest with yourself and see clearly what it is that is motivating you to do what you are attempting. The answer is not always what you think.

Take getting in shape, for example. Many of us will say that the reason we exercise and eat well is to experience greater health benefits. This might be true for some but I'm willing to bet that for many this is actually secondary. The main reason a lot of us exercise and eat well is to look and feel more attractive, whether for ourselves, our partners, or just in general. We train to increase our self-esteem. That is nothing to be ashamed of. You actually sell yourself short by not admitting it to yourself. By being honest and embracing the real reason you are doing something will allow you to get it directly. It will also help you figure out the best way to achieve it, without any fluff or messing around. I know so many women who really want a better bum and legs but they are of ashamed of it. As a result, they keep doing random stuff in the gym in the hope they will materialise one day. Dream on!

As soon as you have your real reason write it down on a piece of paper. By bringing it out of your mind and into the physical world in the form of affirmative words you make it a real thing. Don't believe this will help? Studies have shown that those who write down their goals, as opposed to those who just thought about them occasionally, end up achieving a lot more of the things they want. Write it down and look at it often.

2) Set a deadline

Now that you have a goal fixed firmly in your mind you need to set a deadline for when it will be completed. Leaving important goals on an open timeframe can sometimes be a disguised excuse to not take action. Again, it is a way to avoid the fear and pain of potential failure. Anyone can set a goal and chase it half-heartedly, knowing full well that you are not 100% invested in its attainment. By committing to a set time and date you are breathing real life into your aspirations. They then become a real thing with a lifespan and expiration date. This can be like rocket fuel to your motivation levels.

Ask anybody who functions at a high level or has a demanding job. Setting deadlines makes it far more likely that something will get completed. Deadlines also help us to shuffle our time and to prioritise accordingly. In short, it works, despite the added pressure of a time limit. One of my favourite things to do is to work on my priority goal first thing in the morning, before the rest of the day has a chance to catch up with me. This way I can start my regular routine safe in the knowledge that my main goal is progressing as planned.

Up your level of performance and set rigid deadlines for your goals. If you are true to the process you will be amazed at the results.

3) Identify the enemy

There are not many goals worth having that will just fall into your lap. Despite how we want things to go life will sometimes have other ideas. This will throw all manner of obstacles in your path, many of which you couldn't possibly have planned for.

A great way to cut off any potential obstacles is to make a list of them. Bring them out into the open and become aware of how they might appear. Really use your imagination on this. By imagining all of the unwanted things that might happen, however unlikely, you strip them of the element of surprise. Believe it or not this will make it far more likely that you will stay on course when things get tough. Consider this your mental contingency plan.

Once you have your list go back over it and make a silent commitment to overcome everything on there, if and when it arises. A great technique that I have learned is to actually put yourself on the list. It is hard for us to accept but we are very often our own worst enemies when it comes to achieving our dreams. All of the fears and negative emotions that attack us every day can be the catalyst for failure. We need to become aware of this and to guard our inner space.

You have now looked at the good and bad sides of your goal. You have prepared as much as you can on your own and it is time to bring other people into the plan.

4) Be accountable

The best way to make sure you stick to your goals is to become accountable to other people. This is a stumbling block for some because they like to feel that their goals are personal. There is nothing wrong with this but you are not taking advantage of how our brains are wired. Humans are social creatures and to feel we are moving towards something of value for ourselves and for others is an incredible motivator. Imagine being seen as a huge success in the eyes of your loved ones. For some people this is all they need to burn a lightning quick trail to their most heartfelt desires. It can really light a fuse, as long as the people you bring into your confidence are supportive (choose wisely).

To become accountable, you need to open up to the person or people you have chosen. You need to tell them why you are doing it, what you hope to achieve and when by. The deadline is particularly important. Then, assuming that the person agrees with what you are doing, you need to ask them to keep you accountable. This can mean anything, from weekly progress reports to a daily mail or visit, reminding you to keep going and encouraging you. One of the best ways is to put a monetary price on failure. Offer the other person £100 if you don't follow through and succeed with your goals. They will be more than happy to provide the fuel you need to keep going!

5) Go!

If you follow this process to the letter you will find that setting demanding goals is not the big, bad monster it is sometimes made out to be. Once you have achieved a few things and started to see some real increases in confidence you will actually look forward to setting new goals. The time will almost become a period of introspection or meditation, where you can get back in touch with the things that really matter to you. Especially if you are busy, feeling rushed off your feet and beaten down, goal setting will act as a physical centre and will remind you of where you want to be.

This process is particularly important if you are feeling out of control. Nothing lends perspective and gives you back your power more than reminding yourself you are ultimately in charge. Even five minutes a day focused on your goals can give you the confidence boost you need to go out and meet the world head on. Many times you don't even have to consciously chase your goals. By constant reflection your mind automatically and gently changes course, bringing you into contact with the people and situations that will be able to help the most.

There are other things you can do to enhance the goal setting process, such as producing vision boards full of images of what you would like to achieve. You can also use affirmations and visualisations on a daily basis in order to suggest to the subconscious mind which way you want to go. Personally I have not found these things necessary but many people have. Find out what works for you and does the most to increase your motivation. It is the feeling of unstoppable desire and the thought 'no matter what' that make the most difference. I wish you the best of luck on your goal setting journey.

BREAKING NEGATIVE PATTERNS

How we react to certain situations can mean the difference between success and failure in any endeavour. It's a fact that most of the problems that we encounter in life have their source in our very own reactions to them. If our habitual reflex is to respond in anger, fear, or some other negative attitude, we can be confident that we are only going to exacerbate the issue. This is hard to hear because we never want to believe that we are to blame for something that has gone wrong. On the flip side, it is much easier to play the victim and to give away our power. When we do this we can pretend that everything is out of our control and there is nothing we can do.

Negative thought patterns can have a very corrosive effect on our lives. They can come from anywhere – childhood experiences, parents, work colleagues, siblings, even our partners. At the time you will have no idea that you are adopting something negative, which is what makes it such a slippery and dangerous topic. The effect of persistent negativity in your thoughts, words and actions can have a devastating effect across all major areas of daily life. Relationships can fall apart as the emotional bonds are clouded over by all of the 'bad things'. Work environments can become toxic and alienating if you are always putting things down and voicing issues with other people. Even your personal development can stagnate and regress as you constantly put yourself down.

As a busy mum with a lot of responsibilities I can safely say that I have suffered at times with the quality of my thinking. There is a good chance that you have too. When we find ourselves in the midst of a relentlessly busy schedule that sweeps us along day after day it is sometimes difficult to keep a handle on our thoughts. When our world looks out of control it seems almost natural to throw in the towel internally and spiral downwards too. That's ok. We have all been there. The key is in how you get back up and deal with it.

Falling into habitual negativity is like building a prison around yourself and then throwing the key out of reach. It's a hopeless case, despite the fact we could vanish the prison in a fraction of a second if we really wanted to. It seems so hopeless because a lot of our social conditioning is inherently negative. With so much constant reinforcement going on around us it's easier for us to forget about the self-imposed life sentence and to try and distract ourselves as best as we can. Of course, this only works for a short while. When the movie ends or we have finished that box of cereal we realise we are still in jail and beat ourselves up even more. This turns into a real internal battle and is a key component of Busy Mum Syndrome.

Let's say, for example, that you've noticed you have a habit of thinking negatively about things, especially when you get too busy. Let's also say the situations you get negative about are just normal life challenges that everybody goes through and nobody else seems to get too down about. The issue is in your mind. How do we deal with that?

There are actually a lot of techniques out there that we can use to vanish negative thought patterns. The key premise is that we need to get rid of it entirely and replace it with a new, positive thought so that the old pattern cannot recur. By resisting and beating yourself up about being so negative you actually just reinforce the mental image and make it worse. It makes sense when you think about it – if we use negativity to try and get rid of negativity we are just going to end up with a whole lot more negativity.

Getting rid of these patterns within us can free up a lot of energy that we can put towards our newly set goals from the previous chapter. No matter how overwhelmed you might be feeling right now I speak from experience when I say that it is possible to get things moving in the right direction. With understanding and patience, you can learn to deal with stressful situations from the inside out. As you learn to do this the symptoms of Busy Mum Syndrome will progressively decrease.

Follow this process and get rid of those negative patterns for good:

1) Become aware of specific negative thoughts

Many of us harbour the belief that the negative thoughts we are holding are somehow helping us and saving us from something worse. It is important right from the beginning to change this thinking. All mental and emotional negativity is destructive and unproductive. It serves no direct purpose except to make our muscles tense up and our levels of cortisol to skyrocket, neither of which we want. Once we realise this they lose their value and we can begin to clearly identify thought patterns that recur over time. After this the days of negativity are numbered.

To be more prepared to recognise your negative thinking it is a good idea to know about two of the more common patterns that we all deal with. Doing this will help you to more readily notice where and when your own thoughts turn.

By far the most common negative pattern revolves around anxiety and worry. We worry about everything. Whether it is the car breaking down, the children getting sick or whether we left the oven on, we have a way of turning these thoughts over and over in our minds. Most of what we worry about hasn't even happened and probably won't happen. There is no logic behind anxious thoughts. All we know is that it causes a lot of stress and severely decreases our enjoyment of the moment. Look out for when your mind flings itself into the future in the hunt for something to worry about and gently bring it back to the present. Do not let 'what if' ruin 'what is'.

Another common patterns almost all of us experience is self-criticism. Depending on how much of a perfectionist you are this usually ranges from quite mild to very severe. Many of us are harsh on ourselves because we don't feel like we match up to those around us. We habitually focus on our perceived flaws and weaknesses until that is all we can see. This can sometimes lead to us criticising others as well, which can have the dual effect of destroying our relationships and killing our self-esteem. Mentally beating ourselves up is probably the most useless of all the negative thought patterns. Not only can it drive us in directions we don't want to go, it can also cause us to feel unworthy of love. Listen out for negative self-talk as you go about your day, especially when you feel your stress levels beginning to rise. The quicker we can stamp this out the faster we will feel better and can get started towards our goals.

Negative thought patterns do not have to be focused on the future. They can also come from the past and our previous experiences. If you have felt severe emotional pain in your life there is a good chance you are still experiencing some of the patterns from that time. These can range from feelings of anger and helplessness, to more sophisticated defence mechanisms where we rationalise our reactions and try to assuage some of the guilt. Do not let the past run you. It is long over and holding on to it is only hurting yourself. Have the courage to let it go, as often as you need to, and move forward powerfully.

There are more patterns but these are the three main ones you should become aware of initially. Everyone has their own unique perception of themselves and the world so the chances are your most persistent Fnegative patterns are probably unique to you. Hunt them down ruthlessly and show absolutely no mercy. You will know when you have found one because of the way you feel. Negative thoughts turn your emotions against you, making you feel bad and stripping you of your confidence. Remember that whenever you feel bad you have an opportunity to grow.

2) Select and focus on the positive

Now that you are aware of the dominant negative thoughts in your mind you can consciously begin the replacement process. It is time for you to decide what positive thought you would rather experience. This is an empowering time as you are taking the mental reigns back and regaining control. How long has it been since you did that? Choose a thought that targets a specific negative pattern. Make sure it feels good and makes you feel more confident when you repeat it in your mind. The positive feelings will make the replacement easier and will destroy the disempowering effect of the negative pattern. This bit may take some time to get going but when it does the results are extremely good.

3) Test yourself

Once you have had some success in replacing your negative thought patterns with positive ones it is time to test yourself. This means subjecting yourself to people, places and things that would have sent you into a negative spiral before. You know what they are. All of the things that get your blood boiling and make you want to go back to bed simultaneously. You need to face every single one with the aim to keep your thoughts as positive as possible. If you manage to do this (it may take a few attempts) you will realise something very powerful. You are in complete control of your reactions to the outside world! Nothing can shake you and put you down if you don't let it. All of those negative emotions you have been experiencing, that have been getting in the way of achieving what you want, were completely unnecessary. It is an amazing and frustrating discovery all at the same time. I wish I'd known this earlier!

Practicing in the midst of action like this is the fastest way to make progress. Sports and performance coaches have known for years that thoughts and emotions follow affirmative action. Put another way if you act like you are confident, your thoughts and emotions will catch up and actually produce the feeling of confidence. If you act like you are having the time of your life, very soon your thoughts and emotions will mirror this and you actually will be! It really is an amazing tool that can be used for anything, not just stress management and fitness.

Life is infinitely better when we break our negative patterns, many of which have been running our lives for years without us knowing it. When we make real headway it is almost like there is a disconnect between us and all the things that should make us feel bad. It's as if we know, deep down, that everything will be just fine. It is really a difficult experience to describe so it is best that you find out for yourself.

As we become progressively more positive a few things happen in our lives. Our bodies feel more alive and our minds are more vibrant and creative. Our relationships become amazing and any past resentments or hurts we might have been holding are healed. Our goals no longer look unrealistic or even challenging. We look forward to getting up every day and making meaningful progress towards them, knowing full well that the thing we want is already waiting for us at the finish line. Letting go of negative patterns is like finally taking your foot off the brake. The split second you do it – and a split second is all that it takes – you burst forward and don't look back.

THE MINDFULNESS SECRET: WHAT IT IS, HOW IT WORKS AND HOW TO GET STARTED

Throughout this book we have talked in depth about how to overcome the symptoms of Busy Mum Syndrome. We have, however, neglected to mention one very important topic. Perhaps the most important of all when it comes to mental health and optimal functioning.

Mindfulness is a timeless practice in some cultures and has been for thousands of years. Here in the West it has slowly been catching on since the 1960s and has seen a huge jump in popularity in recent years. This is in no way coincidental with the fact that our lives have become much more fast-paced and, in many ways, out of control. More often than not our minds end up reflecting our external circumstances, which are frequently chaotic. The fact we have turned to ancient practices in order to bring some serenity back to our lives is no surprise at all when you look at it in that context.

For the majority of the population the human brain does not appear to have an off switch. Thoughts bounce around the skull in an endless game, speeding up and blurring together as we get more and more stressed. Then, when you try and stop them, or at least slow them down so you can get some sleep, they rebel and go even faster. You get a headache. Then the alarm goes off.

All we want in life is some positive feelings and a little inner peace.

Chances are you have come across the term mindfulness by now. You may have heard about some of the ways it can reduce your stress levels and help you to relax more. Even medical professionals are recommending it these days so you may have heard it there. If you were doubly stressed that day you might even have downloaded a book on meditation to your iPhone or Kindle and given it a once over. It all sounded great when you started but the only real practical takeaway you got after three hours of reading was to 'observe your breath'. So you tried, once before bed and once again in the morning. You listened and felt your breath for a good twenty minutes before that little voice in your head told you to get up and stop being an idiot. So you did, forgetting all about mindfulness and its supposed benefits. Well it didn't work for me, you find yourself saying. Maybe I'm just not the type.

I promise you right now that you are the perfect person for mindfulness practice. Given a sincere chance it could completely transform your life and the way you see the world. That's because there no 'right' types for mindfulness and meditation. They are perhaps the only true 'one size fits all' remedies in the entire universe. Now, before you throw this book down let me explain. I've been where you are right now. I've sat for hours after a tiring day trying to turn the voice off with absolutely no success. Even when my body was completely finished from training successive clients it would carry on talking like an oblivious relative. At times I felt like I was going completely insane, especially when the meditation practices didn't live up to what had been promised. I gave up time and time again and let the mind take its highs and lows as they came.

Then, one day, it all seemed to click together. Maybe I had suffered through enough practice for the gods of mindfulness to let me into the club. Whatever it was, I realised that I had been forcing my mind to do something it didn't want to do, which was causing it to act up even more. When I allowed it to do what it wanted – which is actually the art of mindfulness – it threw its toys out of the pram for a while but eventually quietened down enough for me to gain some clarity. I had found something that works! I tried it throughout the day and it worked there too. The increase in peace and wellbeing was noticeable from the start and only got deeper. My daily activities became easier, more patiently attended to and even joyful.

Learning the things that I did I believe you can have the same, if not a deeper, experience. How? We'll get to that. First let's back up and talk about what mindfulness actually is.

Mindfulness is essentially paying attention to something – a kind of non-judgemental interest where we observe without thought. The intention has to be to let the mind rest on the object of attention for a prescribed period of time, without forcing it to. This is the real trick to success in this practice because the mind will rebel against anything that you 'force' it to do. The key is to keep your attention wide open and relaxed, as if there is nothing you would rather be doing in the world. When your interest becomes genuine – and it will do, given time – the mind will cease to wander too much and you will find a peace that you may never have experienced before. Even so, when it does wander, as it will do in the beginning, gently regain control of your focus. Don't be harsh on yourself. There is absolutely no right or wrong way here. It is all in how the practice makes us feel.

I recommend that you use this 'open interest' method in solitude to start with. Shut the door and turn your phone off for ten or twenty minutes. If needs be wake up a little earlier or go to bed a little later if that is all of the quiet time that you have. At first, when your mind is liable to jump all over the place at the slightest thing, this will work much better if you have no distractions. Later on, when your mind has quietened down to the point where you don't feel like you are at its beck and call anymore, you can practice this method anywhere and everywhere. We will talk about how to do this now.

Think about all of the things that you do during the day. Taking and picking up the kids from school. Driving to and from work. Taking a shower. Doing the dishes. Going to dinner with your spouse or partner.

Now think about all of the times you feel stressed or experience negative feelings during the day. I bet there are many more stresses than activities! Well, what if we could do all of these things in a mindful way? What if we could take the inner peace we have been cultivating in our quiet times and make it a day-long experience?

The good news is that we can and, if you have been putting the solitary work in, the transition is easy. The key to doing it is to fully open up your awareness as you have been doing. Have a mild, non-judgemental interest in everything that you do. This is a form of equanimity, an essential virtue in Buddhism. If your mind wanders or you feel a part of the body contract you know it is the beginning of the stress mechanism. By keeping your awareness open at all times this becomes very easy to spot. When this happens bring your attention gently to your five senses. Make an effort to really feel what you are feeling, smell what you are smelling, and hear what you are hearing. Feel the movement of our body as you direct it, notice the energy flow up and down your spine. Remember that the senses can anchor you in the present moment and use them to that purpose when you are struggling to maintain open awareness in your daily life.

The benefits of using this method are numerous. For one, open awareness knows no boundaries or places it can't go. You can use this method at work, when driving, when shopping or training in the gym. Nothing is exempt from inner peace and, as your practice grows stronger, you will find that it permeates everything that you do, even situations that you would have found very stressful in the past. At times the peace will be so profound you can't help but laugh and sit back, feeling gratitude for everything you have been through so far. At other times it will be a powerful undercurrent, quietly reminding you everything is ok when external things seem to be falling apart.

Another benefit is a rapid increase in confidence and the realisation that you can handle whatever life throws at you. If that person shouts at me, it's ok. If things don't go to plan that is fine too. You can't really put a price on this. Don't worry if you find yourself contracting still after a few months of practice. These mechanisms are deeply imbedded in the human psyche and will take a fair amount of time to root out completely. Holding the intention, however, guarantees that it will be done.

Mindfulness practice should never be complex or demand too much mental work. It should never feel like a chore or something that we have to do. A big help is to remember that the majority of our thoughts are absolutely useless, with no practical value at all. If we were to look at the contents we would see 40% worries, 30% babble and 10% regrets, leaving only 20% that is actually of use in our day to day existence. You will be doing them and you a favour by taking the reins back and quietening them down. Taking control back from the mind is one of the most empowering things you can do in life. When you do you find yourself giving less attention to the past and the future and far more to the present moment. If you have painful or traumatic memories in your past, like most of us do, this will make you want to laugh out loud and shout from the rooftops. Realising that you are not the often negative thoughts and feelings that pervade our consciousness is an extraordinary discovery. If it makes you feel good I suggest you do it. That's what it is all about, after all.

For many people lasting inner peace and joy is seen as an unattainable goal. This is because they have been tricked by their own thinking into believing it so. Ever noticed how the mind tries to keep us focused outward, filling us up with desires for so many things we don't know which way to turn? That's because it doesn't want us to look within. It doesn't want us to realise the thoughts and feelings we suffer through on autopilot are actually optional. That most of them get in the way of doing, being and having a lot of what we want. The thing is that mindfulness is not hard at all. As a practice it is essentially devoid of effort, once the initial awareness has been established. We must commit to staying open and allowing whatever life turns up with without withdrawing in on ourselves. This will feel so weird at first because it seems as though we are more vulnerable than usual. For once, perhaps for the first time in our lives (definitely since childhood), we have intentionally set our guards down and are discovering the world as if it is new. This is such a powerful thing to do. After the initial trials of staying open to things that we normally turn our backs on we find ourselves in place where we can barely be hurt. Our energy system re-aligns spontaneously and we find ourselves far more assertive, confident and creative than ever before. Your enthusiasm for everything skyrockets! Family and friends start to notice and ask you what you are doing differently. Random people in the street look at you in a funny way, as if you have something they need. It's crazy. Honestly, I'm excited for you.

BRINGING IT ALL TOGETHER

In this last section I want to leave you with some motivational words that I hope will help you on the journey. As a busy mum, I know that getting in shape physically and mentally can be a tough road, especially without any prior knowledge or support. I want you to know that I am here for you every step of the way.

Making a commitment to yourself to getting back into shape is one of the best investments you can make. The simple act of seeing yourself in the mirror, exactly as you would like to be, is so transformative that it is hard to put into words. You will have to experience it for yourself to see what I mean. Don't let anything stop you until you do.

Education is key. If you are just starting off or have made a commitment to take your health seriously there are worse things to spend your money on than expert advice. Saying that there are a lot of top-notch free resources out there on the internet for both training and nutrition, many of which you can find at **kellyrennie.com**.

Ultimately, getting our diet and exercise in check is just one way to shift the dial of our lives in a positive direction. The other way is to look after your mind and to be grateful for what you have every day. I know I am.

In this book we have talked about everything you need to begin your journey to a happier, more inspired life as a busy mum. I hope the lessons will help you as much as they did me, through the good times and bad, as we all move closer to achieving the goals we set for ourselves.

I am looking forward to hearing about your successes in the near future.

You can find me at:

www.busymumfitness.com

Facebook: https://www.facebook.com/kellyrennieBusyMum/

Twitter: https://twitter.com/kellyrennie

Instagram: https://www.instagram.com/kellyrenniefit/

Feel free to hit me up at any time with your questions and we will work through this together!

Thanks,

Kelly

WOULD YOU DO ME A FAVOUR?

A huge, huge thank you for buying my book. I hope you enjoyed it and found the information valuable. I wholeheartedly believe that if you absorb and apply what you have read you will find yourself looking and feeling better than you have done in years.

    Now that we know each other better I have a tiny favour to ask. Would you take two minutes out of your day and leave some feedback for this book wherever you purchased it? I read all of my reviews and love to get feedback. It also helps to get the word out, which allows me to keep helping people ☺

    Thankyou!

Printed in Poland
by Amazon Fulfillment
Poland Sp. z o.o., Wrocław